SECOND EDITION

HANDBOOK FOR NEWLY DIAGNOSED CASES OF ADHESIVE ARACHNOIDITIS

Steps for Treatment

By
Forest Tennant, DrPH, MPH, MD

Published by Arachnoiditis Hope
Tennant Foundation
West Covina, California

SPONSORS OF THIS BOOK
Tennant Foundation
336-338 S. Glendora Ave.
West Covina, CA 91790-3043
Ph: 626-716-2689
Fax: 626-919-7497
Email: tennantfoundation92@gmail.com

ISBN: 9781955934480
Library of Congress Control Number: 2025912299

Special discounts are available on quantity purchases by corporations, associations, educators, and others. For details, contact one of the parties listed below.

U.S. trade bookstores and wholesalers: Please contact Nancy Kriskovich Tel: (406)249-2002;
or email snkriskovich@gmail.com

All proceeds from the sale of this book will go to Arachnoiditis Hope sponsored by the
Tennant Foundation
336-338 S. Glendora Ave.
West Covina, CA 91790-3043
Ph: 626-716-2689
Fax: 626-919-7497
Email: tennantfoundation92@gmail.com

Arachnoiditis Hope Acknowledgements

Medical Director

Martin J. Porcelli, DO, MPHF, PhD

Research

Ingrid Hollis

Publication

Nancy Kriskovich

Podcast

Jaime Sanchez, RN

Website and Bulletins

Rebecca Cholcher-Marino

Table of Contents

Author's Notes

Arachnoiditis (ARC) Hope was initiated about eight years ago to bring diagnosis and treatment of ARC to every community. Over this period, we have conducted several studies, analyzed over 2000 magnetic resonance images (MRI), and reviewed hundreds of AA cases. Adhesive arachnoiditis (AA) of the lumbar spine and non-adhesive arachnoiditis of the cervical spine are the problematic clinical diseases that cause the most misery and pain. This is the second edition of "Handbook for Newly Diagnosed Cases of Adhesive Arachnoiditis." It is primarily directed at persons who have recently been diagnosed with AA, but it can also be instructive for persons who have cervical ARC and persons with AA who aren't doing well.

AA is an inflammatory/autoimmune disease of the arachnoid membrane and cauda equina nerve roots which are in the lower spinal canal. Effective treatment requires a three-component protocol: (1) suppression of inflammation and autoimmunity, (2) regeneration of damaged nerve tissue, and (3) control of pain. To accomplish these measures, one must systematically build a therapeutic treatment program. It is our clear belief that if any of the steps given in this handbook are skipped or ignored, effective control of AA will likely be elusive.

Since I started Arachnoiditis Hope, I've observed that "Hope" has constantly been forthcoming. I've now observed "too many to count" persons with AA who have controlled the "devil's disease" and now lead a quality life.

Introduction

Adhesive arachnoiditis (AA) is a progressive inflammatory/autoimmune disease of the arachnoid membrane and the cauda equina nerve roots. History has clearly told us that this disease may progress to paralysis, incontinence, a bed-bound state, and early death if not controlled. The rate of disease progression varies from person to person. For example, the time between disease diagnosis and paralysis or a bed-bound state can vary from weeks to years. The major goal of this handbook is to help newly diagnosed cases of AA start a treatment protocol that will halt AA progression. In order to accomplish this goal, some specific steps must be initiated. Once stability is achieved, there are measures that some persons with AA have successfully used to reverse symptoms and complications and even achieved "near cure."

It is essential that one knows some basic facts about the arachnoid membrane. It is the inner lining of the spinal canal cover. The outer layer is called "dura," and it is thicker and tougher than the arachnoid, which is thin and fragile. The arachnoid membrane has a "spiderweb-like" appearance when viewed under a microscope. Its functions are to structurally support the dura, regulate spinal fluid, and provide nutrition for the dura and other spinal canal tissues. When injured due to a tear, infection, or inflammation, it is very painful. If inflamed or infected, it may cause cysts (e.g., Tarlov's) or spinal fluid leaks. Inflammation of the arachnoid membrane is simply called "arachnoiditis." It is a common cause of pain associated with herniated discs, spinal stenosis, and failed back surgery syndrome.

AA occurs when an inflamed arachnoid membrane produces glue-like adhesions and fuses with cauda equina nerve roots. The inflammation, adhesive process forms micro-masses inside the spinal canal that entrap nerve roots which connect and regulate the functions of the legs, feet, intestine, bladder, and sex organs. The inflammatory, adhesive process causes great erosion and damage to both cauda equina nerve roots and arachnoid membrane.

The micro-masses impede normal spinal fluid flow. Unless controlled, paralysis and neurologic dysfunctions will eventually occur in the legs, feet, bowel, bladder, and sex organs. Severe, chronic pain, debilitating fatigue, weakness, impaired mental function, and shortened life span will also occur without adequate treatment. Due to these severe complications, we advocate that every person with AA take a stepwise, systematic approach and build a solid therapeutic program rather than simply thinking that pain relief, a good night's sleep, or some single curative measure is all that is needed.

Adequate treatment requires a three-component protocol:

(1) suppression of inflammation and autoimmunity
(2) regeneration of damaged nerve tissue
(3) control of pain.

This handbook will give you enough information and options to administer the three-component protocol. We also caution persons with AA who believe they can skip steps or an entire component of the protocol. Our experience after reviewing several hundred AA cases is that relief, recovery, comfort, and a quality of life depends on executing all three protocol components.

Exclusions

The therapeutic measures provided in this handbook are primarily for persons with AA who are ambulatory, have no severe neurologic impairments, and can carry out activities of daily living. The therapeutic measures provided here may not be applicable to persons with late-stage AA who are not ambulatory, have significant neurologic impairments, and are bed or house-bound. In these cases, palliative measures may be more appropriate rather than the treatment recommendations in this handbook.

Inclusions

The measures and steps in this handbook may be applicable to those ambulatory persons who have been given the diagnosis of:

1. Non-adhesive arachnoiditis
2. Chronic cauda equina inflammatory disorder
3. Cervical arachnoiditis

Therapeutic Steps

Step One: Keep Doing What Works

Except for direct trauma and injury to the spine and spinal canal, AA does not happen "overnight." It is always the end result of multiple medical diseases, events, and complications. The pathologic process necessary for the development of AA may range from months to years.

During the pathologic run-up to AA, you undoubtedly have attempted many medicinals. These likely include prescription and non-prescription medications for symptoms such as pain, lack of sleep, weakness, energy, and motivation, among others.

Review an inventory of every medication, vitamin, mineral, and herbal/natural supplement you take. Keep taking any and all that you perceive to help. Also, any diet exercise, or other measure that reduces pain or helps you function should be continued.

In summary, build your protocol starting with medications and measures that have already worked for you.

Step Two: Put Together Your Medical Records

AA doesn't just happen. It is the end result of multiple other medical conditions and pathologic events that may have taken place over several years. You may have a genetic or childhood disease that initiated your path to AA. Since AA is a serious, unusual disease, you will need a hand-carry set of life-time medical records to show all medical parties you encounter. These may include your insurance company, pharmacy, and hospital.

We highly recommend you obtain photographic copies of the MRI images that document you have AA. Attached is a list of the eight major symptoms of AA. Rarely does a person with AA have less than four major symptoms. Check the symptoms you have and put it in your permanent, hand-carry medical records. Your records should also contain any laboratory and other medical tests that document your medical history.

Some of the medications that you will need to treat AA may likely be subject to regulations and laws. To satisfy regulations you may have to document you have AA. Persons who believe that their records are safely kept and easily accessible at a medical facility or stored in a phone or computer may find that treatment for AA is not forthcoming. Most medical practitioners today won't wait for stored records that may or may not show up for days or weeks. In summary, have a hand-carry medical record that documents you have AA.

	Eight Major Symptoms of Adhesive Arachnoiditis	Y	N
1	Sharp, stabbing pains in your lower back, buttocks, or groin/crotch area when you twist, turn, or bend		
2	Bizarre skin sensations such as crawling insects or water dripping down one or both legs		

3	Burning pains in your feet and/or groin/crotch area		
4	Your pain temporarily lessens when you stand or recline		
5	Leg weakness		
6	Pain that radiates down one or both legs		
7	Bladder dysfunction that may include dribbling, urgency, or difficulty starting or stopping urination		
8	Head or cerebral symptoms which may include headache, vertigo, dizziness, or blurred vision		

Note: Persons who have four or more of the major symptoms listed here almost always have adhesive arachnoiditis.

Step Three: Determine Your Likely Causes

There are some genetic diseases, traumatic events, infections, autoimmune diseases and other conditions that may occur early in life and put a person at high risk to develop AA in later life. The attached Table lists these risk factors. One risk factor requires immediate attention. There is a genetic connective tissue disease known as Ehlers-Danlos Syndrome (EDS) that is highly associated with AA. Many persons who have developed AA are unaware they have this condition. Attached is a screening test to help you determine if you have Ehlers-Danlos Syndrome (EDS) or another related connective tissue disorder. If you score high on the attached screening test for connective tissue disease, make sure your medical practitioners are aware of this fact.

The basic causes of AA fall into one of two categories:

1. Direct injury to the arachnoid membrane by trauma, infection, toxic contaminant in spinal fluid, or electrocution.
2. Inflammatory, autoimmune disease that originates outside the spine and eventually causes inflammation in the arachnoid membrane.

	Screening Test for Ehlers-Danlos Syndrome	Y	N
1	Do you have pain in multiple locations?		
2	Do you have extreme fatigue?		
3	Are you clumsy sometimes and fall or walk into objects?		
4	Are some of the joints in your hands, feet, elbow, hips, or knees "loose" or quite flexible?		
5	Have you had a lot of sprains or joint dislocations?		
6	Is your skin thin in places?		
7	Are you double-jointed or able to bend your fingers, arms, or ankle backward?		
8	Are your hands and feet cold much of the time?		
9	Do you bruise easily or have bruises that suddenly occur?		
10	Is your skin "stretchy" in some places?		
11	Are you constipated a lot?		
12	Do you suffer from "heart burn" or frequent episodes of food regurgitation?		

If you answer yes to six or more of these questions, you likely have Ehlers Danlos Syndrome (EDS).

Persons who develop AA due to injury of the arachnoid membrane are normally well-aware of the accident, infection such as meningitis, or industrial or other accident that may have contaminated spinal fluid with a toxin or caused electrocution. Today, most persons who have AA develope it as a result of an autoimmune, inflammatory disease that originates outside the spine. A traumatic event such as an epidural injection, especially in a person with risk factors, may trigger AA.

Our studies have identified some risk factors that make one more prone to develop AA. It may occur due to a precipitating event that "kicks off" the disease. Both the major risk factors and precipitating events for AA are shown here. There are some AA cases, however, in which no precipitating event seems to have occurred. Persons who are in this category usually start with mild back pain that progresses into severe back pain along with other major symptoms of AA.

TABLE
Risk Factors and Precipitating Events for AA

Risk Factors[+]

A. Genetic Connective Tissue Disorder (Examples: Ehlers-Danlos or Marfan Syndrome)
B. Spinal, Anatomical Abnormality (Examples: Scoliosis, Spondylolisthesis)
C. Autoimmune Disease (Examples: psoriasis, rheumatoid arthritis, ankylosing spondylitis, systemic lupus, viral reactivation)
D. Severe infection in the past (Examples: Lyme, infectious mononucleosis, meningitis, pneumonia)
E. Severe trauma or accident (Examples: vehicle, domestic, combat, fall, sports, electrocution)
F. Two or more of the following medical disorders: herniated discs, sciatica, migraine headache, carpal tunnel, fibromyalgia, irritable bowel, thyroiditis, small fiber neuropathy, arthritis, myalgiaencephalopathy/chronic fatigue syndrome (ME/CFS)

Some Precipitating Events*

A. Spine or head trauma from a fall or accident
B. Medical procedure including surgery, spinal puncture, epidural injection
C. Acute infection; viral or bacterial

+Risk factor means a pathologic condition or event that makes one more likely to develop AA than other people.

*Some persons don't appear to have a precipitating event but develop AA over time usually as a result of a slow or mild autoimmune disorder.

Step Four -Start a Daily Protein, Anti-inflammatory Diet

AA is a progressive, degenerative disease caused by chronic inflammation. A diet with daily protein and anti-inflammatory foods is basic to control the disease. Protein contains the amino acids that regenerate nerve tissue including the arachnoid membrane. It also makes the neurotransmitters such as endorphin and dopamine as well as some hormones that control pain. AA may cause a loss of appetite and taste so persons may reject a lot of foods and liquids. The key is to settle on a daily diet that you will follow. Given the distortion of normal appetite by AA, the usual strict do's and don'ts of most diets are not recommended for AA. Attached are Tables that show the common protein and anti-inflammatory foods, so you can pick and choose.

You will most likely need to reduce your carbohydrate (sugars) intake. Your blood sugar (glucose) must not be allowed to rise to high levels which will occur with high carbohydrate foods such as breads, regular sodas, pastry, pasta, and candy. High blood sugar promotes inflammation. The attached Table shows some tips on keeping down blood sugar levels. Many persons with AA report benefit in reducing gluten in their diet, so you may wish to eliminate it.

Collagen and/or amino acid supplements are popular with AA persons. We have seen no difference between effectiveness of powders, bars, drinks, or capsules. Furthermore, we do not know of a standout brand. A collagen or amino acid supplement is highly recommended if you can't eat protein foods each day.

The Basic AA Daily High Protein, Anti-Inflammatory Diet

1. Each day: eat one or more of these protein foods: beef, lamb, pork, poultry (chicken, turkey), seafood (fish, shrimp, crab), cottage cheese, eggs

2. Each day: eat some vegetables and/or fruits

3. Stop drinks that contain regular sugar (carbohydrates) including fruit juices, soft drinks, coffee, and tea

4. Restrict sugars and starches known as carbohydrates (e.g., breads, candy, pastries, pasta, pizza)

5. Low amounts of alcoholic beverages are permitted

Table of Some Common Protein and Anti-Inflammatory Foods	
Protein Foods	Some Anti-Inflammatory Vegetables/Fruits
Seafood: Fish, Shrimp, Crab Beef Pork Lamb Poultry: Chicken, Turkey Eggs Cottage cheese	Broccoli Green beans Leafy greens: Spinach, Lettuce, Kale Peas Corn Blueberries Apples Oranges Pineapple Grapes Watermelon Cantaloupe

At least one serving of protein and anti-inflammatory foods is required each day.

Step Five: Hydrate (Drink Fluids) Every Two Hours

AA is an inflammatory disease of the lower spinal canal. Inflammation in tissues produces heat, electricity, and damage. In the process, it also produces toxic waste products. Unless removed by spinal fluid, the inflammatory waste increases the inflammatory assault on the arachnoid membrane and cauda equina nerve roots. Drinking enough fluids during waking hours is a key to removal of inflammatory waste in the spinal canal.

About 500 milliliters of spinal fluid are made each day to keep adequate spinal fluid in the canal. New spinal fluid is made about every four to six hours to keep the canal full of fluid and keep it moving up and down the spinal canal. Besides carrying out inflammatory toxic waste, it also carries out viruses and brings in nutrients and medications. Imagine a creek or stream half full. Stagnation, toxins, and vegetation take over. The same principal applies to the spinal canal.

Spinal fluid is made from the fluids one drinks. Sickness such as AA tends to dissipate a desire to eat and drink. Consequently, think of liquids including water, sodas, coffee, or other as medicine. If it is liquid and you swallow it, the body will take part of it and make spinal fluid.

Our strong recommendation is to drink a liquid every two hours while awake. It may only be a few swallows, but setting a regular schedule of every two hours will most likely provide the body enough liquids to maintain normal levels of spinal fluid.

Step Six: Start Select Vitamins and Minerals

There is a group of vitamins and minerals that assist all three protocol components. While a daily multi-vitamin-mineral tablet or capsule may have benefits, they don't usually have a high enough dosage of any one ingredient to accomplish the needs of an AA patient. The basic vitamin/mineral supplements listed here are to assist suppression of inflammation and autoimmunity, regenerate damaged nerve tissue, and reduce pain. In addition, the vitamins and minerals listed here are known to help prevent reactivation of the Epstein-Barr Virus.

<u>Vitamins</u>

Vitamin C, 2000 mg in AM and PM
Vitamin B-12, 500 to 1000 mg daily

Vitamin D, 500 to 800 units a day

<u>Minerals</u>: Magnesium, selenium, zinc, boron

A person with AA is well advised to use more than one mineral. Take one of the minerals each day. They can be rotated.

Step Seven: Spinal Fluid Flow Exercises

Spinal fluid is renewed or "changed over" like oil in a crank case about every 5 to 6 hours. Spinal fluid is a critical body component. It carries nutrients and medicinals to spinal canal tissues including the cauda equina and arachnoid membrane. Equally or more important is that it carries out all toxins, organisms, and metabolic waste that may accumulate in the spinal canal in order to keep the spinal fluid clean, nutritious, and capable of healing. We recommend some special exercises to keep the fluid moving.

The arachnoid membrane is "avascular" in that it has no blood supply. It depends on spinal fluid to bring it essential nutrients and medications. A medicine, in order to be effective in treating AA, must enter the spinal fluid rather than rely on the bloodstream.

The micro-masses of AA impede spinal fluid flow. Certain physical exercises will accelerate or enhance the flow to improve healing and prevent the complication of impaired spinal fluid flow.

Here are Common Clinical Complications from Blockage or Impairment of Spinal Fluid Flow:

Spinal fluid leaks	Nasal/eye watering	Fainting/falling
Tinnitus	Headaches	Vertigo
Increased cranial pressure		

Given here are exercises to enhance or accelerate spinal fluid flow. They are simple and some should be done at least once or twice each day by persons with AA to promote healing and prevent complications.

Spinal Fluid Flow Exercises

1. Rocking chair – 5 to 10 minutes
2. Walking or gentle bouncing on a trampoline – 3 to 5 minutes
3. Porch swing, 5 to 10 minutes
4. Deap breathing – hold 30 seconds; repeat 5 to 10 times
5. Arm swings while walking

Do one or more of these exercises each day.

Step Eight: Wear A Back Brace During Waking Hours

If you have MRI-documented AA, you will need to wear a back brace during waking hours. AA is always accompanied by one or more degenerated spinal tissues that may include intervertebral discs, vertebrae, facets, and ligaments. AA entraps cauda equina nerve roots in an adhesive, inflammatory mass. Essentially all persons with AA have one or more degenerating discs that have slipped and press against the canal cover which is composed of the dura and arachnoid membrane. Persons who have had surgery or have scoliosis or spondylolisthesis put extra strain on inflamed tissue. All in all, a person with AA has a very unstable back and will likely deteriorate and develop more pain and impairment unless their spine and back get extra support that only a back brace can provide.

One small, sudden jerk or movement in a person with AA can cause a tear of either the arachnoid membrane or cauda equina nerve roots. This can come about when one suddenly jerks, falls, or only has a mild stumble while walking. Bending over is a risk to persons with AA. A brace and a slow bend will protect you.

Selecting a Brace: Go to a pharmacy, sporting goods store, or medical supply outlet. Most carry a variety of back braces. Select a soft, flexible brace. Try it on at home. Make sure it is comfortable, supportive, and will fit under your clothes.

Make the Brace a Clothing Item: Let's face it. No one likes to wear a brace, but with AA you have no real choice. Far too many persons with AA have had a stumble or jerk and experienced a permanent setback. Put the brace with your clothing and consider it a part of daily attire. You get dressed every day and now you simply have an additional piece of clothing called a brace.

A Plus for a Brace

Many persons with AA have reluctantly started to wear a brace but were pleasantly surprised that the brace significantly reduced their pain.

Chronic Deterioration

A back brace isn't just to protect you from a sudden fall, jerk, or stumble. It is to primarily keep you "straight" or "in balance." Simply leaning or favoring one side or the other, overtime, will lead to chronic friction and deterioration of spine tissues. The following schemata show how degenerated discs and entrapped nerve roots can lead to increased pain and neurologic impairments.

Schemata of How a Slipped Disc Presses and Scrapes the Arachnoid Membrane

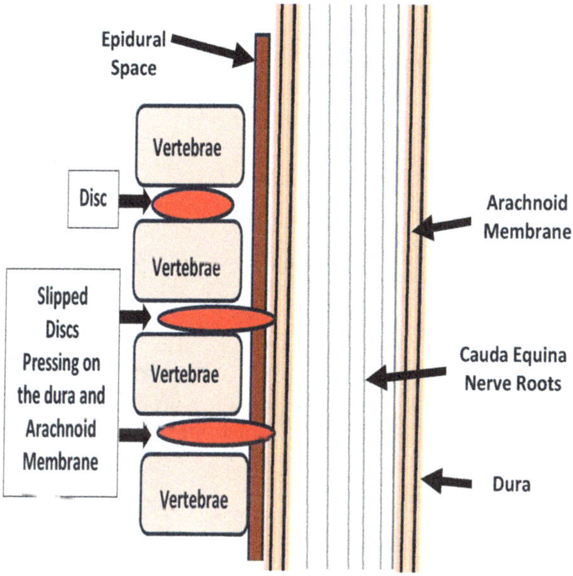

As a person moves or especially jerks or bends, the discs scrape and inflame the arachnoid membrane. Discs that degenerate and press upon the arachnoid membrane are inflamed, and they spread inflammation to the arachnoid membrane.

Diagram of Entrapped Nerve Roots in AA

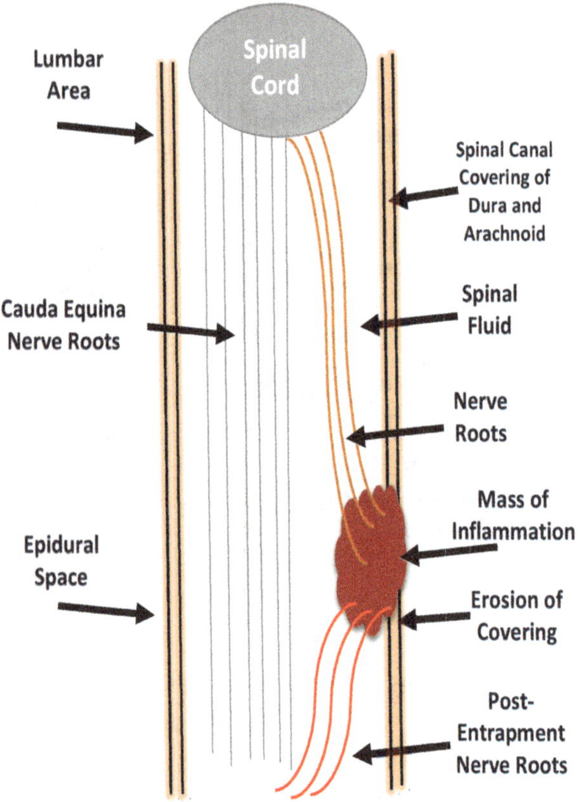

The entrapped nerve roots must continually activate the legs, feet, bowel, bladder, and sex organs. Over-stretching or jerking can tear the mass and permanently injure a nerve root. A brace may prevent this from happening.

Hopefully treatment can dissolve adhesions. Treatment of AA attempts to prevent scarring and calcification of the mass so that the nerve roots will remain alive, functional, and prevent permanent neurological impairments.

Step Nine: Wear Snug, Supportive Shoes

The previous step described how a brace may prevent a twist, jerk, or fall from injuring the arachnoid membrane or cauda equina. To also prevent injury, it is necessary to wear supportive shoes. Footwear such as sandals, open back slippers, high heels, or loose loafers will simply not adequately prevent stubbed toes, jerks, and falls. Except while in bed, the proper, safe shoes are tie-ons or snug slip-ons.

Step Ten: Don't Sit Over 30 Minutes

The most common spinal canal location for AA micro-masses is around the lumbar five and sacral one joint. This location puts pressure on the micro-masses of AA when one sits. If one feels pain when sitting, it means you are squashing cauda equina nerve roots, and you need to immediately stand. Many persons with AA have learned the hazard of sitting for an extended period while in a car or airplane or sitting and watching a good TV show. Some have foolishly continued to sit even after pain started and caused increased neurologic damage.

To keep from squashing an inflamed AA micro-mass, one needs to refrain from sitting more than 30 minutes at a time. After 30 minutes or even sooner if pain starts, stand and preferably take a short walk with some deep breathing. Stand for at least a few minutes.

Reclining doesn't usually harm the micro-masses of AA. Lying on a flat surface spreads the pressure over a wide area rather than does sitting.

Step Eleven: Begin Regenerative and Recovery Exercises

AA, if uncontrolled, can be progressive and produce paralysis of feet, legs, bladder, bowel, and sex organs. It may leak or seep spinal fluid into the muscles and supporting tissue just outside the spine. In the latter case, chronic seepage can permanently constrict back muscles that connect to the arms and legs causing extension to be restricted.

Nerves, including those in the cauda equina may heal and regenerate, if used, while lack of use may cause degeneration ("use it or lose it"). In AA the recurrent and habitual use of arms, legs, and feet will help prevent deterioration and regenerate cauda equina nerves. Listed here are critical exercises some of which a person with AA must do to not only prevent deterioration but promote regeneration.

Walking: Walking is the physiologic cornerstone of AA nerve regeneration. Persons with AA need to take at least two short walks a day (at least 100 feet). Walking upstairs or on a treadmill is excellent.

Extend and Flex: Next to walking, fully extending one's arms and legs at least half a dozen times a day is essential. Flexing arms and legs can follow or precede extension. Ankle and foot flexing, while either sitting or standing, should be done several times a day. Knee raising and holding for 2 to 3 seconds can be done sitting or standing. This can be done several times a day.

- ✓ Extend arms overhead and from side to side.
- ✓ Stand and extend one leg at a time.

- ✓ Stand and raise each knee for 5 to 10 seconds.
- ✓ Flex your ankle and feet several times a day.
- ✓ Stand and rock back and forth on your toes and heels several times a day. (May need to hold onto a chair or cabinet while doing this.)

Weightlifting: Lifting a 2-to-5-pound weight is highly recommended twice a day. Simply raising the weight to your body (curls) and raising the weight overhead done on a regular basis will strengthen muscles and other tissues around the lower spine. We believe that light weightlifting done daily will strengthen spinal ligaments and spinal canal cover as well as the arachnoid membrane.

In summary, the recommended regeneration exercises are walking, extending and flexing extremities, and light weightlifting. Keep body parts "fidgeting" and moving every day.

Cautionary Notes:

1. Physical therapy by therapists who aren't keenly aware of AA is risky. Many persons have been permanently damaged by overly aggressive therapists and chiropractors. Please warn all therapists of this fact.

2. No exercise should cause pain or fatigue. Stop any therapy or exercise that elicits pain.

Step Twelve: Identify Some Topical Pain Relief Measures

The pain that accompanies AA may emanate from both inside the spinal canal and in the soft tissues surrounding the spine. These tissues include muscle, fascia, connective tissue and skin.

Pain from inside the spinal canal comes from inflammation and tissue damage to the arachnoid and cauda equina. Unfortunately, arachnoid membrane inflammation may cause erosion of the spinal canal cover so seepage or leakage of spinal fluid may occur. Spinal fluid is a toxic, painful irritant to tissue outside the spinal canal.

After a diagnosis of AA is initially made or during a painful episode in a person with an established diagnosis, an attempt should be made to relieve pain by topical ("rub-on") application of a medication. Every person with AA should identify at least one or two topical or rub-on treatments.

To start, go to a pharmacy and obtain some "BioFreeze" and "Lidocaine." Both come as rub-ons, sprays, and patches. One or both will usually provide some back pain relief, particularly if there is spinal fluid seepage into tissues around the spine.

There are various pain patches including "Salonpas™" and others. See if one will provide relief. The same goes for herbal drops and creams such as boswellia, aloe vera, and arnica.

Magnet and copper rubs may be helpful. Some authorities claim this to be placebo. We disagree based on the many positive reports we receive about this centuries old practice.

An old-fashioned heating pad should be tried. Also, there are inexpensive infrared and electromedical devices (Example: TENS) on the market that should be tried. Recently some lasers and what are called pulsed energy devices have come on the market at a reasonable price. At this time, we don't have a favorite brand, but as this handbook is being written, we have many positive reports about a number of devices. Persons with AA should try these devices as they have no serious side-effects and may provide relief and regeneration of nerve tissue.

In summary, a person who has recently been diagnosed with AA has to identify some local and topical back pain relief measures. They will likely have to be used in the future for flares. You may identify some measures that not only provide relief but some permanent recovery.

Step Thirteen: Water Soak Each Day

Over the centuries water soaking (hydrotherapy) has been practiced and observed to heal and relieve pain. This age-old practice is quite applicable to AA. We recommend a daily soak.

The term "water soaking" usually conjures the belief that you must immerse yourself in a pool or jacuzzi. While soaking up to your neck in water is an ideal therapy, water soaking simply means that you expose your back to water. Here is a list of water soaking measures that can be used by a person with AA:

1. Stand in a shower and let water flow off your back, neck, and legs.

2. Immerse your body up to your neck in a bathtub, hot tub, jacuzzi, or pool.

3. Drape a warm, water-soaked towel over your back.

4. Soak your feet and ankles in warm water.

The above soaks can be done from 5 to 15 minutes. Minerals or herbs can be put in foot baths. One long-standing and popular mineral preparation is Epsom Salts.

Why does water soaking have a therapeutic effect? Two common beliefs are:

1. Water relaxes muscles and increases blood flow to the damaged areas of the body.
2. Water extracts excess bioelectricity that has accumulated due to inflammation

and damage to the neurologic circuitry in the body.

Step Fourteen: Start Medical Treatment With Natural/Herbal, Non-Prescription Medicinals

The medical protocol to treat and control AA requires three components: (1) suppression of inflammation and autoimmunity, (2) regeneration of damaged nerve tissues, and (3) control of pain. Initiating this protocol doesn't require a medical professional.

AA is a rare or unusual disease, so as of yet, there are no physician specialists. A person with AA may have a delay or difficulty finding a physician who will prescribe and treat AA. Consequently, we strongly urge persons with AA to initiate treatment with non-prescription, natural, herbal medicinals as soon as possible. Please recall that AA is a progressive disease, so no time should be wasted to start the three-component medical protocol. Physician prescriptions can be added at any time to non-prescription medicinals.

Listed here are our current recommendations. They have been selected as they have, to date, been the most popular with persons who have AA. The non-prescription medicinals recommended are to be continued along with any prescription drugs prescribed by a physician.

Natural and Herbal Medicinals to Start the Three-Component Medical Protocol

1. Suppression of Inflammation and Autoimmunity Initially select one, but two can be obtained and rotated on different days. Follow the labeled dosage instructions: serrapeptase, quercetin, astragalus.

2. Regeneration of Damaged Nerve Tissue: Dehydroepiandrosterone (DHEA). Dosage is 100 to 200 mg a day

3. Control of Pain: palmitoylethanolamide (PEA) Dosage is 300 to 600 mg twice a day (PEA). It can be in addition to other pain relievers. Some PEA products are enhanced with luteolin or other herbal agents. They are most acceptable.

Unfortunately, persons with AA may find it difficult to find a prescribing physician, or they may find that their physician provides minimal help. In this situation, persons with AA may have to mostly "self-treat." Listed here are some non-prescription options or add-ons to the basic, three-component medical protocol given above.

Pain Relief and Nerve Tissue Regeneration

Peptides: a. BPC-157
b. Thymosin

Pain Relief and Inflammation Suppression

a. Chinese skull cap with other ingredients (TH-1 Support™) or other
b. Lion's mane mushroom extract
c. KAVA
d. Kratom
e. CBD/marijuana
f. Mucuna
g. St. John's wort

Natural Hormones for Pain Relief and Nerve Tissue Regeneration

a. Whole adrenal gland
b. Colostrum
c. Deer/elk antler extracts

Step Fifteen: Consult Your Personal Physician

Once you have gone through the steps listed here and started the three-component medical protocol, consult your personal physician. Take all of your medical records and a summary of the steps you have already taken to build an effective treatment program.

Shown here is the starting three-component medical protocol we suggest that utilizes prescription drugs. Show it to your medical practitioner as he/she will have to decide what fits the requirements and limitations of their practice.

Starting Medical Protocol with Prescription Drugs
Suppression of Inflammation and Autoimmunity
Diclofenac, 50 to 75 mg a day in divided dosages, or extended release 100 mg
Regeneration of Damaged Nerve Tissues
Medroxyprogesterone, 2.5 mg three times a week - oral
Control of Pain (Choice of one)
1. Low dose naltrexone 2. Buprenorphine 3. Tapentadol 4. Hydrocodone or oxycodone with acetaminophen
Notes for Medical Provider
1. The above Table lists our recommendations to initiate medical treatment with prescription drugs for a newly diagnosed case of lumbar-sacral adhesive arachnoiditis. 2. Elsewhere in this handbook, patients are encouraged to initiate treatment with non-prescription medicinals. They can be continued with prescription medications. 3. Any previously prescribed effective pain relief medication should be continued. 4. This starting regimen should be re-evaluated at 60-days.

Step Sixteen: Establish a Daily Treatment Routine

During your first 60 days following diagnosis of AA, you should establish a daily routine of the steps and therapeutic measures given here. Consistency is a major key to controlling AA. One can and should continuously try to enhance their daily program.

We wish to point out that many persons with AA make the mistake of believing that they can skip some of the steps given here. For example, a common misconception is a belief that exercises, and suppression of inflammation, aren't important, so they skip them and only rely on pain relief.

One must constantly keep in mind that AA is a progressive inflammatory, autoimmune disease that can suddenly and unexpectedly cause paralysis, dementia, and total debilitation. To best insure this won't suddenly happen to you, execute the full three-component medical protocol as part of your regular daily routine.

The Sixty-Day Evaluation

The 60-day evaluation of a patient with adhesive arachnoiditis (AA) should categorize the patient into one of these two basic classes:

1. Unstable:
    a. Pain is poorly controlled and interferes with normal physical and mental functions and activities of daily living.
    b. Urination impairments are present
    c. Leg/foot burning, shooting pains, and sensations of crawling insects or water dripping are present
    d. Blurred vision, vertigo, tinnitus, or migraine are present

   e. Walking requires assistance or is uncomfortable
   f. Cannot fully extend arms and legs

2. Stable:
   a. Pain is controlled enough to preserve physical and mental functions and carry out activities of daily living
   b. Urination is normal or has only minor symptoms
   c. Leg/foot burning, shooting pains, and sensation of crawling insects or water dripping have improved or resolved
   d. No blurred vision, vertigo, tinnitus, or migraine present
   e. Can walk without assistance or discomfort
   f. Can fully extend arms and legs

It is recognized that the two categories may have some overlap, but one category will be prominent. Persons who are unstable will require additional pain control measures. These can include raising the dosage of opioids or adding medicinals directed at neuropathic pain (Examples: gabapentin, pregabalin, diazepam), or descending pain (Examples: tizanidine, clonidine, methylphenidate, amphetamine salts, dextroamphetamine). Another option is to initiate a weekly dose of: (1) ketorolac (10 to 30 mg), and (2) methylprednisolone (4 mg).

Persons with AA who have stabilized should initiate measures that may reverse symptoms and the pathologic process of AA. There are now many persons with AA who have achieved "near cure." Measures for stabilized cases can include the addition of the polypeptides BPC-157 and thymosin. Anabolic hormones including human chorionic gonadotropin, progesterone, or testosterone are popular. Breakup of AA micro-masses seem to have occurred in some patients by use of pentoxifylline or the administration of electrical currents and/or electromagnetic energy waves.

All persons with AA at the 60-day evaluation should ideally have blood panels for hormone levels and Epstein-Barr virus antibodies. The hormone panel consists of cortisol, pregnenolone, testosterone, and dehydroepiandrosterone (DHEA). Estradiol and progesterone are optional. Any low levels indicate that replenishment should be done. Testing for Epstein-Bar Virus (EBV) antibodies is to determine past and present reactivation and autoimmunity. Recent research has shown that EBV, often in conjunction with other viruses, may accelerate or worsen AA by either infiltration of the arachnoid membrane and cauda equina nerve roots or by an autoimmune process that erodes these two tissues. EBV reactivation may be the cause of AA instability and deterioration, and control measures, depending on test results, must be initiated.

Summary

AA is an inflammatory, autoimmune disease that is fusion of the arachnoid membrane and cauda equina nerve roots in the lower spinal canal. Regardless of the underlying causes and precipitating factors of AA, there are basic therapeutic measures that must be part of a treatment program.

We highly recommend that the basic treatment steps described in this handbook be systematically incorporated into a daily therapeutic program. Once basic treatment measures have been initiated and stability has been established, additional treatment measures for AA should be attempted.

Glossary of Terms in this Handbook

Adhesive Arachnoiditis: An intraspinal canal inflammatory disorder in which there is a clump or mass of cauda equina nerve roots that are fused by adhesions to the arachnoid-dural covering of the spinal canal.

Arachnoiditis-Non-Adhesive: Inflammation of the arachnoid layer of the spinal canal covering without any nerve roots adhered to it. This condition cannot specifically be identified by MRI. It is a clinical diagnosis based on signs, symptoms, and laboratory tests.

Ascending Pain: Pain that occurs due to transmission of bioelectricity from the site of nerve injury or dysfunction up through the spinal cord into the brain.

Cauda Equina: Nerve roots that emanate from the spinal cord at about the level of thoracic 12(T-12) or lumbar 1 (L-1) and are suspended in spinal fluid.

Centralized Pain: Constant pain that results when glial cells become dysfunctional.

Central Sensitization: Pain perception that is excessive for the injury that produces the pain. It is caused by dysfunction of glial cells.

Clumping or Coalescence: Multiple nerve roots have joined together due to inflammation and adhesion formation.

Connective Tissue Disorder: A genetic disease in which collagen in tissues deteriorates, weakens, and subsequently develops inflammation and pain in the tissues. The most common is Ehlers-Danlos Syndrome (EDS).

Corticoid or Corticosteroid: A pharmaceutical that is chemically related to cortisone.

Descending Pain: Pain that occurs due to transmission of bioelectricity from the brain down the spinal cord and vagus nerve.

Epidural Injection: An injection given in the space just above the spinal canal.

Lumbar Spine: A lower back section of the spine consisting of five lumbar vertebrae levels being designated L1 through L5 with L1 being the topmost vertebrae.

Meninges: This is the covering of the brain and spinal cord that primarily consists of an inner layer called pia mater, middle called arachnoid, and an outer layer called the dura. The word "covering" is preferentially used in this handbook rather than meninges or theca to simplify understanding.

Neuropathic Pain: Pain that occurs when transmission of bioelectricity is impaired or blocked in the brain, spinal cord, or peripheral nerves by a disease or injury.

Sacral Spine: The lowest section of the spine usually consists of three vertebrae. These vertebrae are designated S1, S2, and S3.

Spinal canal: The spinal canal is a structure like a closed pipe that contains the spinal cord and contains spinal fluid. The fluid is primarily produced in the brain and flows down the canal on one side and flows back up to the brain to be diverted into lymph nodes and the general body, blood and lymphatic systems. The word canal is preferentially used here to simplify understanding. The lower spinal canal is sometimes called "thecal sac."

Spine: Refers to multiple tissues including vertebrae, intervertebral discs, spinal canal, cord inside the canal, and cauda equina nerve roots.

Spinal Tap: A puncture of the spinal canal to either place a substance inside the canal or withdraw fluid.

Medical References

1. Aldrete JA. History and evaluation of arachnoiditis: The evidence revealed. *Insurgentes Centro 51-A. Col San Rafael, Mexico* 2010; p3-14.
2. Aldrete JA. Suspecting and diagnosing arachnoiditis. *Pract Pain Mgt* 2006;16:74-87.
3. Aldrete JA. Arachnoiditis: the silent epidemic. *Future Med Publishers, Mexico* 2003.
4. Anderson TL, Morris JM, Wald JT, et al. Imaging appearance of advanced chronic adhesive arachnoiditis: A retrospective review. *Am J Roentgenol* 2017;209:648-655.
5. Andre G, Trompet E, Snoeck R. Novel therapeutics for Epstein-Barr virus. *Molecules* 2019;24:997-1009
6. Bilello J, Tennant F. Patterns of chronic inflammation in extensively treated patients with arachnoiditis and chronic intractable pain. *Postgrad Med* 2016;92:1-5.
7. Bjornevik, et al. Longitudinal analysis reveals high prevalence of Epstein-Barr virus associated with multiple sclerosis. Science 2022 DoI:10.1126/science.abj8222.
8. Burton C. Lumbosacral arachnoiditis. *Spine* 1978;3:24-30.
9. Castori M, Voermann NC. Neurological manifestations of "Ehlers-Danlos Syndromes. *Iran J of Neurol* 2014;13:190-208.

10. Coronel MF, Labomlorda F, Roig P, et al. Progesterone prevents allodynia after experimental spinal cord injury. *J of Pain* 2011;12:71-83.
11. Dawson-Basoa M, Gintzler AR. Estrogen and progesterone activate spinal kappa-opiate receptor analgesic mechanisms. *Pain* 1996;64:608-615.
12. Delamarter RB Ross JS, Masaryk TS, et al. Diagnosis of lumbar arachnoiditis by magnetic resonance imaging. *Spine* 1990;15:304-310.
13. DiSanto E, Fodde MC, Ricciardi-Castognol P, et al. DHEAS inhibits TNF production in monocytes, astrocytes and microglial cells. *Neuroimmunomod* 1996;3:285-288.
14. Djeball M, Guo Q, Pertus EH, et al. The neurosteroids progesterone and allopregnanolone reduce cell death, gliosis, and functional deficits after traumatic brain injury in rats. *J Neurotrauma* 2005;22:106-118.
15. Eisenberg E, Goldman R, Schlag-Eisenberg D, et al. Adhesive arachnoiditis following lumbar epidural steroid injections: A report of two cases and review of literature. *J Pain Research* 2019;12:513-518.
16. Epstein NE. The risks of epidural and transforaminal steroid injections in the spine: commentary and a comprehensive review of the literature. *Surg Neurol* 2013;4(supp2):574-593.
17. Frye CA, Duncan JE. Progesterone metabolites, effective at the GABA(A) receptor complex, attenuate pain sensitivity in rats. *Brain Res* 1994;643:194-23.
18. Harley JB, et al. Transcription factors operate across disease loci, with EBNA2 implicated in autoimmunity. *Nat Genet* 2018;50:699-707.

19. Harrow T. Epstein-Barr virus could be a cause of multiple autoimmune disorders. *VA Research Currents* April 18, 2018.
20. Hamonet C. Ducret L. Ehlers-Danlos, an Unknown and Disturbing Syndrome. Free Comments. *Theranostics Brain, Spine & Neural Disord* 2017,2:555-591.
21. Henderson FC, Austin C, Benzel E, et al. Neurological and spinal manifestations of the Ehlers-Danlos Syndromes. *Amer J Men Gen* 2017;175C:195-211.
22. Horsley V. Chronic spinal meningitis: its differential diagnosis and surgical treatment. *Br J Med* 1909;1:513-517.
23. Jackson A, Isherwood I. Does degenerative disease of the lumbar spine cause arachnoiditis? A magnetic resonance study and review of the literature. *Brit J Radiology* 1994;67:840-847.
24. Jakhmola S, Jha HM. Glial cell response to Epstein Barr Virus infection: a plausible contribution to virus-associated inflammatory reactions in the brain. *Virology* 2021;559:182-195.
25. Jones KJ. Gonadal steroids and neuronal regeneration: a therapeutic role. *Adv Neurol* 1993;59:227-240.
26. Jorgenson J, Hansen PH, Steenskoo V, et al. A clinical and radiological study of chronic lower spinal arachnoiditis. *Neuroradiology* 1975;9:139-144.
27. Karishma KK, Herbert J. Dehydroepiandrosterone (DHEA) stimulates neurogenesis in the hippocampus of the rat, promotes survival of newly formed neurons and prevents corticosterone induced suppression. *Eur J Neurosci* 2002;16:445-453.

28. Kerr J. Epstein-Barr virus (EBV) reactivation and therapeutic inhibitors. *J Clin Pathol* 2019;0:1-8.
29. Kiefer, et al. Effects of dexamethasone on microglial activation in vitro. *J Neuroimmunology* 1991;34:99-108.
30. Kiguch et al. Chemokines and cytokines in neuroinflammation leading to neuropathic pain. *Curr Opinion Pharmacol* 2012;12:55-61.
31. Lei ZM, Rao CV. Neural actions of luteinizing hormone and human chorionic gonadotropin. *Seminar Reprod Med* 2001;19:103-109.
32. Loggia MI, Chunde DB, Oluwaseum A, et al. Evidence for brain glial activation in chronic pain patients. *Brain* 2015;138:604-615.
33. Nagata K, Hayashi K. Epstein-Barr virus reactivation-induced immunoglobulin production: significance on autoimmunity. *Microorganisms* 2020;8:1875-1890.
34. Parenti V, Huda F, Richardson PK, et al. Lumbar arachnoiditis: Does imaging associate with clinical features? *Clin Neurol Neurosurg* 2020;192:105717.
35. Quiles M, Marchiselo PJ, Tsairis P. Lumbar adhesive arachnoiditis: Etiologic and pathologic aspects. *Spine* 1978;3:45-50.
36. Reddy DS. Neurosteroids: endogenous role in the human brain and therapeutic potentials. *Prog Brain* Res 2010;186:13-137.
37. Rodriguez LJG, Sandoval Sanchez V, Benavides Rodriguez D, et al. Paraplegia due to adhesive arachnoiditis: a case report. *Act Ortop Mex* 2009;23:232-236.
38. Roglio I, Bianchi R, Gotti S, et al. Neuroprotective effects of dehydroeprogesterone and progesterone

in an experimental model of nerve crush injury. *Neurosci* 2008; Aug 26;155(3):673-685.

39. Sevesto S, Merli P, Ruggier M, et al. Ehlers-Danlos icSyndrome and neurological features: a review. *Childs Neuro Syst* 2011;27:365-371.
40. Sotkin ML Riella G, Formaglio F, et al. Central effort of ketorolac involving MDA receptors activity. *Brain Res* 1998;223-226.
41. Takahashi H, Suguro T, Okazima Y, et al. Inflammatory cytokines in the herniated disc of the lumbar spine. *Spine* 1996;21:218-224.
42. Takedo, et al. Effect of methylprednisolone on neuropathic pain and spinal glial activation in rats. *Anesthesiology* 2004;100:1249-1257.
43. Tennant F. Human chorionic gonadotropin in pain treatment. *Prac Pain Manag* 2009;9:25-27.
44. Thomas J. Arachnitis and Arachnoiditis. *Comprehensive Medical Dictionary. Philadelphia, J.B. Lippincott & Co.* 1873;p57.
45. Tsuda M. Microglia in the spinal cord and neuropathic pain. *J Diabetes Investig* 2016;7:17-26.
46. Webster KM, Wright DK, Sun M, et al. Progesterone treatment reduces neuroinflammation, oxidative stress and brain damage and improves long-term outcomes in a rat model of repeated mild traumatic brain injury. *J Neuroinflammation* 2015;18:12-238.
47. Whendon JM, Glassey D. Cerebrospinal fluid stasis and its clinical significance. *Altern Ther Health Med* 2009;15:54-60.
48. Wood RA, et al. Serologic markers of Epstein-Barr virus reactivation are associated with increased disease activity, inflammation, and interferon

pathway activation in patients with systemic lupus erythematosus. *J Translational Autoimmunity* 2021;4:1000-117.

49. Zang Y, Chee A, Shi P, et al. Intervertebral disc cells produce interleukins found in patients with back pain. *Am J Phys Med* 2016;95:407-415.

Index

<u>OTHER BOOKS BY FOREST TENNANT</u>

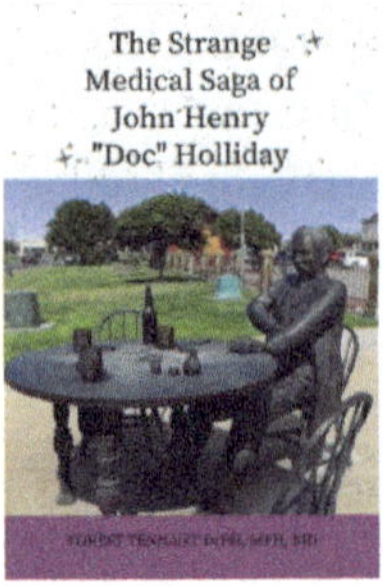

The Strange Medical Saga of "John Henry"

ISBN: 9781955934275
LOC: 2023913628

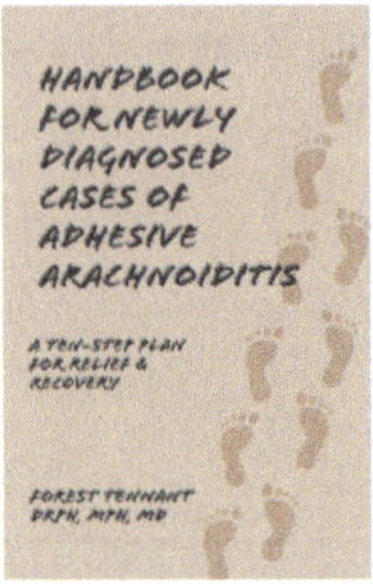

Handbook For Newly Diagnosed Cases of Adhesive Arachnoiditis

ISBN: 9781955934244
LOC: 2023908116

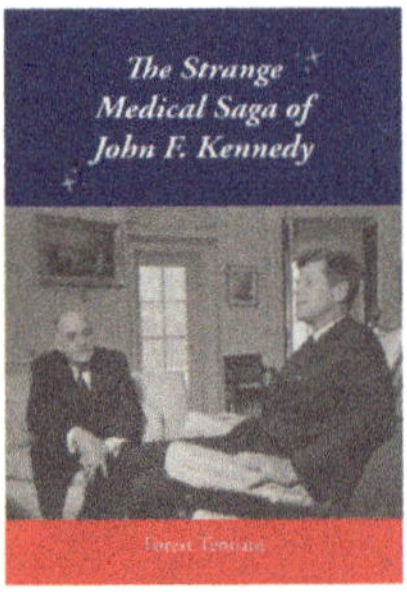

The Strange Medical Saga of JFK

ISBN: 9781955934213
LOC: 2023903440

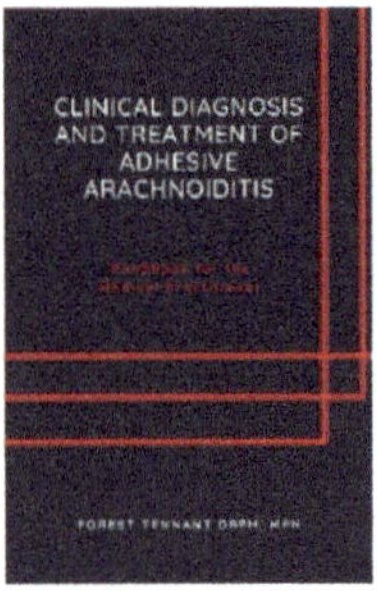

Clinical Diagnosis and Treatment of Adhesive Arachnoiditis

ISBN: 9781955934183
LOC: 2022907190

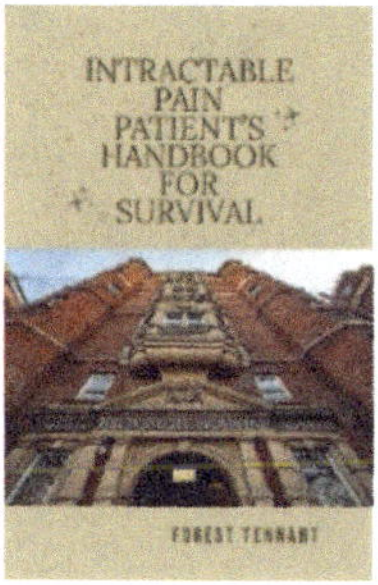

Intractable Pain Patients Handbook for Survival

ISBN: 9781955934121
LOC: 2021916464

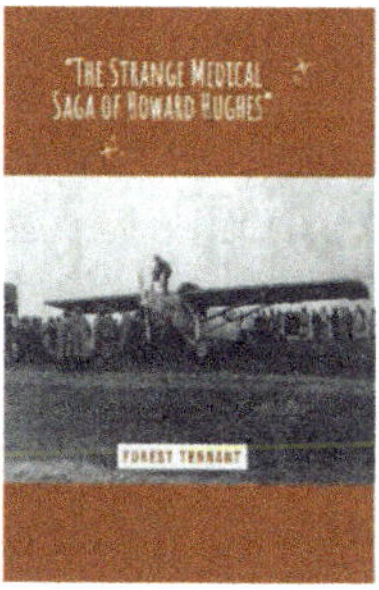

The Strange Medical Saga of Howard Hughes

ISBN: 9781955934091
LOC: 2021912855

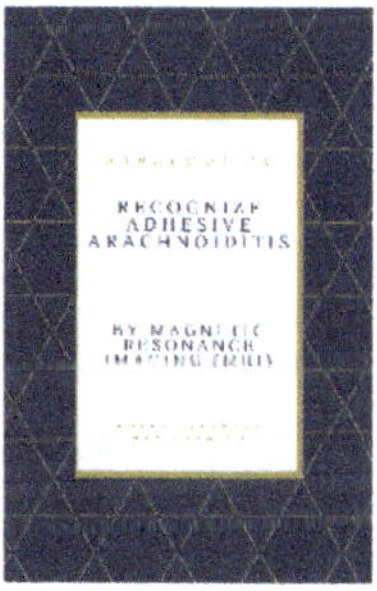

Handbook To Recognize Adhesive Arachnoiditis by Magnetic Resonance Imaging (MRI)

ISBN: 9781955934152
LOC: 2021925161

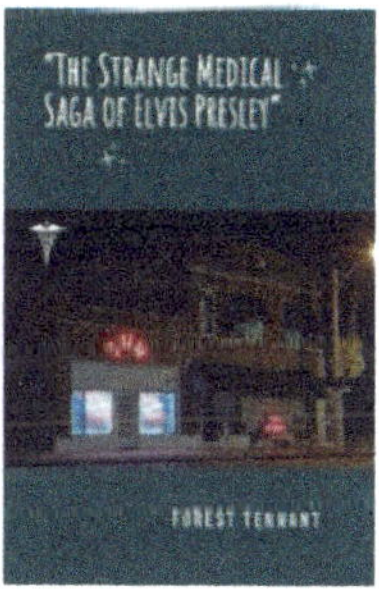

The Strange Medical Saga of Elvis

ISBN: 9781955934008
LOC: 2021911718

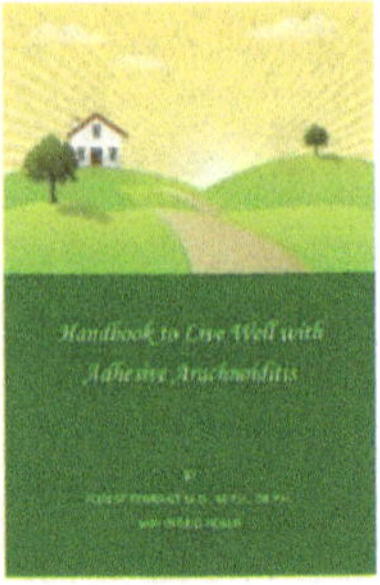

Handbook to Live Well with Adhesive Arachnoiditis

ISBN: 978195934060
LOC: 2021912718

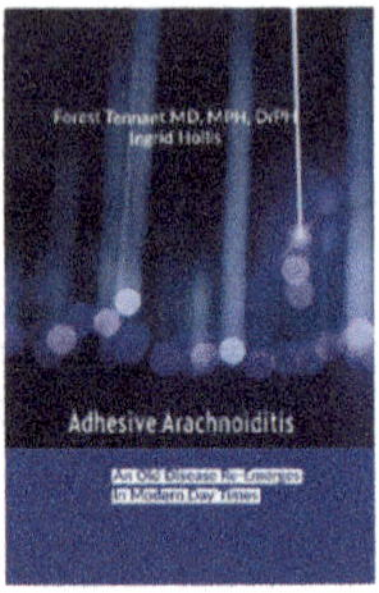

An Old Disease Re-Emerges in Modern Times

ISBN: 9781955934039
LOC: 2021912467

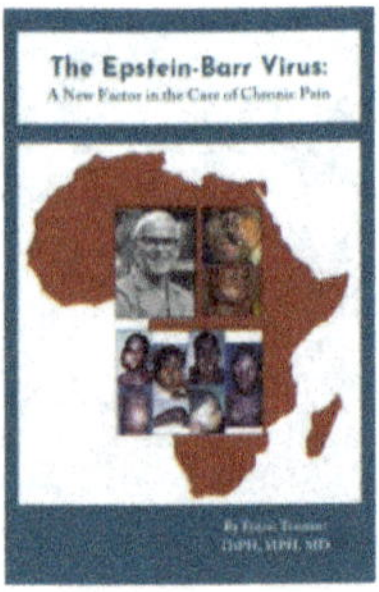

The Epstein-Barr Virus: A New Factor in the Care of Chronic Pain

ISBN: 9781955934428
LOC: 2024919179

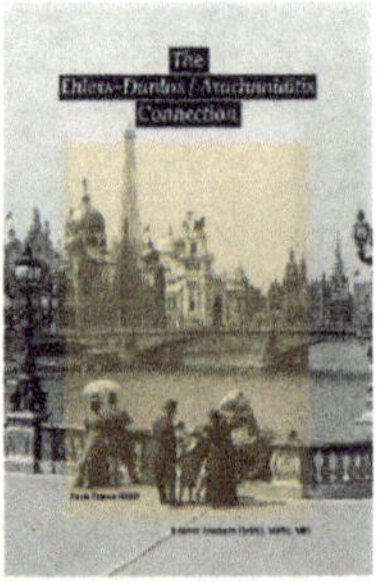

The Ehlers-Danlos / Arachnoiditis Connection

ISBN: 9781955934381
LOC: 2024911409